MAN'S SEXUAL ENRICHMENT FORMULA

For the prevention and treatment of erectile dysfunctions (ED), also known as "Impotence", sexual urge booster, penis enlarger, and energy & stamina enrichment.

Dr. Inks Swiss

Table of Contents

Copyright Notice. By Dr. Inks Swiss

Introduction

MEN'S SEXUAL ENRICHMENT FORMULA" is a complete natural male sex enrichment formula that is very active in the prevention and treatment of numerous kind of erectile dysfunctions such as; poor sexual urge or desire, poor libido premature ejaculation etc. and also, if you are having issues satisfying your partner in bed because you are having small penis and you want to enlarge it to become harder and tougher.

Do you desire to be energetic, enhance your stamina and endurance to achieve a long lasting erection?

What are you still waiting for? Why not CLICK THE BUY BUTTON and experience an ever electrifying and amazing sex life that your partner could ever imagine!

CHAPTER ONE
ENRICHMENT FORMULA
What Is MEN'S SEXUAL ENRICHMENT FORMULA?

MEN'S SEXUAL ENRICHMENT FORMULA is a natural male enrichment formula that is formulate stimulate your body natural ATP to enhance or boost the Nitric Oxide production and also stimulate vasodilatation, which on the other hand, will lead to addition of the quantity or rate of blood that will flow down direct to the chamber of the penis and stir the arteries in the penis for stronger and tougher erection.

What Are The Benefits Of MEN'S SEXUAL ENRICHMENT FORMULA?

The benefits of MEN'S SEXUAL ENRICHMENT FORMULA are:

1. This natural enrichment formula can help you to enhance your stamina and endurance level to

achieve a long lasting sexual activity with your partner

2. MEN'S SEXUAL ENRICHMENT FORMULA can help you to gain a potent stronger and bigger erection that will stay longer

3. With it potential qualities of natural active solution which is very essential in the body that assist nitric oxide stimulate the boost of blood flow to your penis

4. It can also help you to regain your sexual urge and self-confidence to your sexual lifestyle

5. It can help you stay in charge of your sexual activities with your partner

6. MEN'S SEXUAL ENRICHMENT FORMULA helps you to boost your orgasm to enjoy electrifying love making with your spouse

i. MEN'S SEXUAL ENRICHMENT FORMULA gives you superb gains & energy. Therefore, you will heighten your sexuality and relationship.

CHAPTER TWO
Complete Review Of MEN'S SEXUAL ENRICHMENT FORMULA
What Are The Advantages Of MEN'S SEXUAL ENRICHMENT FORMULA?

The advantages of MEN'S SEXUAL ENRICHMENT FORMULA are:

1. MEN'S SEXUAL ENRICHMENT IS FORMULA is formulated with the best 100% natural ingredients that helps in enhancing men sexual overall performance

2. Is a very safe supplement that can help you boost your sexual activities without any side effects

3. If after 60 days of consumption of this supplement and you didn't get your anticipated result you can return it as it guarantee money refund.

4. It can be ship all over the world and shipping fee is free

5. When you begin to administer this supplement you don't need to change your regular diet

6. Trust me with MEN'S SEXUAL ENRICHMENT FORMULA your anticipated result for consumption is sure

7. Since it is 100% natural formulated, this supplement don't require a physician prescription

8. It can also be used to edify your entire mood

9. It is well package in a plain way that not even your spouse will have an idea of what you have ordered.

Disadvantages Of MEN'S SEXUAL ENRICHMENT FORMULA

The disadvantages of MEN'S SEXUAL ENRICHMENT FORMULA include:

1. Some time it might take a longer period of time to get your anticipated result due to different body system

2. It can only be order from the manufacturer website.

Why do I need MEN'S SEXUAL ENRICEMENT FORMULA?

The reality is that in every ten men in the world one suffers

from erectile dysfunction, so you don't have to let your be

the one people that could be suffering from ED out of this ten men, which is the actual reason why you need this superb supplement to help reshape your sexual lifestyle again. This supplement is different from other supplement that initiate deceitful chemical reaction that don't stay long will boost the interaction of two energy system in your body called the ADP & ATP; this can help your body refurbish its vivacity, strength, energy, stamina and endurance level to enable you enjoy a long lasting sexual period with your spouse.

The Citrus and Pomegranate used in the making of this superb supplement would help to enhance the ATP that already exist in your body allowing you to enjoy additional energy when required and also increase the Nitric oxide in your body system helping you to benefit from vasodilation, and when the flow of blood is improved your circulation too increased because the arteries smooth muscle are relaxed, as a result of this, it allows your muscle organs and penis to retain more blood to make you gain and sustain a good erection that will result to an outstanding orgasm.

The horny goat weed that is added in the making of this superb supplement contain an active ingredient known as the icarin- which is a prenylated flavonied constituent that helps to block a protein related with erectile dysfunction called the PDE5.

Gingko is also added to improve oxygen supplies to the body, by breaking down platelets that assist flow of blood to the entire body easily and broadening the vessels that carry blood into the brain. However, ingesting MEN'S Sexual Enrichment Formula will help to enrich the brain sexual sense functionality and entire blood circulation in the body.

Another included constituent known as Tribulu Terrestris that is added in the making of MEN'S SEXUAL ENRICHMENT FORMULA is a natural herbs that is usually recommended for men health because of its qualities that it contains to increase libido, vivacity, vigor strength erectile dysfunction (ED) and testosterone production. These are all the health benefits that you stand to enjoy when you ingest MEN'S SEXUAL ENRICHMENT FORMULA.

CHAPTER THREE
How Does MEN'S SEXUAL ENRICHMENT FORMULA Works to boost Erection?

For you to really know how active MEN'S SEXUAL ENRICHMENT FORMULA works to enhance erection you will first of all know what erection is or what bring about erection. To get an erection you must be sexually aroused, the nitric oxide in your body will make the muscle of corpora cavernosa to be calm permitting more blood to flow into the open space. The blood will now build pressure in the corpora cavernosa allowing the penis to expand however creating a stronger and tougher erection.

This superb supplement include the best quality constituent in the world that can help your body naturally boost its ATP and Nitric Oxide proficiency, both which are very vital for enhancing the blood flow and boosting mitochondrial action, everything that you desire to stimulate a steady, bigger, larger and tougher erection. Therefore, once you are a regular consumer of MEN'S SEXUAL ENRICHMENT FORMULA, you are certain of a greater erection that will result to extreme orgasm.

Who is MEN'S SEXUAL ENRICHMENT FORMULA Formulated For?

MEN'S SEXUAL ENRICHMENT FORMULA this man effective formula is not out there for everyone, below is a group of individuals that this superb man formula is meant for: male potency formula is not meant for everyone, here is the list of people this cutting-edge male formula is meant for:

i. This constituent is put together to help those who has already loss confidence in their self and can no longer be in control of their sexual session with their partners.

ii. This formula is made for man who are willing to

restore their sexual pleasure or stimulation

iii. This constituent is made for those individuals who desire to be in charge of his bedroom

iv. Is for those individuals who find it very hard to sustain hard long lasting erection when needed

v. This constituent is required by individuals that lack the strength, vivacity and energy to satisfy his spouse sexual desire

vi. Is formulated for that man who desire to improve his stamina and endurance level to stay longer in his sexual session with is partner

vii. Is for those individuals out there who are suffering from erectile dysfunction (ED) and required 100% nature treatment for it

viii. It is for those individuals out there who are willing to enhance their mental and physical performance in the gym

ix. This constituent is made for those men out there who desperately want to boost their sexual drive and libido

x.   This constituent is carefully formulated for those individuals out there who need fast and active male natural enrichment formula without no side effects

xi.   It for those man who desire to intensify their orgasm

CHAPTER FOUR
What Are The Required Dosage of MEN'S SEXUAL ENRICHMENT FORMULA?

MEN'S SEX ENRICHMENT FORMULA male this effective's formula usually comes inside a box and each of this boxes contains 10 tablets. You are required to ingest 1 tablet 30 minute before you engage in your sexual session to enable you achieve maximum anticipated result. The moment that you ingested this supplement, instantly you will be begin to experience multiple benefit like blood vessel dilation, enhanced circulation and so much energy, this will enable you get harder, tougher, thicker long lasting erection, revitalized libido, extreme stamina & endurance level etc.

However, it is strongly advisable to give yourself space from consuming MEN'S SEXUAL ENRICHMENT

FORMULA every three to four month interval for your body system not to get addicted or use to the supplement. This is because consuming the supplement for a very long period of time might cause your body to be immune to the effect of MEN'S SEXUAL ENRICHMENT FORMULA.

What Are The Safety Measures of Consuming MEN'S SEXUAL ENRICHMENT FORMULA?

The precautions of consuming MEN'S SEXUAL ENRICHMENT FORMULA are:

i. Keep the supplement in a cold place away from moisture and light

ii. All supplement should be well protected from children

iii. Women should stay away from this supplement for they are not supposed to ingest this supplement

iv. Any person below the age of 18 are not are not supposed to use this supplement

v. Please don't ingest more than a tablet as

recommended

vi. Please if you are allergic to any of the constituent that is use in the making of this superb supplement don't ingest it

vii. Please ensure you consult your doctor if you are precisely undergoing any medication before you using the supplement

viii. If you are having any health history or medical condition please you ensure you talk to your doctor before using this supplement

ix. It is recommend to be ingested 30 minute before you engage in your sexual activity

x. If the seal of this supplement is found damage in anyways don't consume it

What Are The Possible Side Effects I Can Experience From Consuming This Supplement

Although MEN'S SEXUAL ENRICHMENT FORMULA is usually recognized with no side effect however the side effects under-listed are rare cases recorded from few of the consumers, but you should note that if you carefully follow the recommend dosage trust me you might not experience any of this side effects:

i.   Stomach discomfort

ii. Vomiting

iii. Headache and

iv. Nausea

This potent male effective formula is manufactured by Swiss Research Labs

CHAPTER FIVE
What Are the Potential Ingredients Use in the Making of MEN'S SEXUAL ENRICHMENT FORMULA?

MEN'S SEXUAL ENRICHMENT FORMULA is a 100% men performance formula which contain the following constituent:

i.   Horny goat weed

ii.   Tribulus terrestris

iii.   Pomegranate

iv.   Ginkgo Biloba

v.   Panex Ginseng root

vi.   Citrus sinensis

vii.   Zinc

viii.   And other ingredients

What Is Horny Goat Weed?

Horny Goat weed also called barrenwort or fairy wings is a flowering plant in the family of Berberidaceae whose lot of the species are consider rampant to Asia, China and Mediterranean region. It is also known as the "Natural Viagra" because of its many useful qualities like aphrodisiac properties, enhanced testosterone production, enhancing memory functions, bone and kidney health.

The name Horny goat weed was generated when a Chinese shepherd discovered that anytime his goat feed on the flower plant they sustain a long lasting erection during intercourse, that is to say the goat become sexually stimulated with so much energy.

Horny goat weed is known to have a very strong active component referred to as icarin this is a flavonoid ingredient that aid to increase the affirmative function of

Nitric oxide in the body.

The expected benefit of Horny Goat weed are:

i. It can increase your lean muscle mass and also increase your energy level

ii. It plays a very vital role in prevention of bone loss and minimizing of cartilage degradation in people suffering from Osteoarthritis

iii. It aids the circulation of blood in the body

iv. It aids male ability to get and sustain erection because it triggers flow of blood to the penis

v. This natural Viagra aids to block the protein connected to ED

vi. It can used for the treatment of premature ejaculation and poor libido

vii. Horny goat weed also aids to enhance liver function

viii.   Horny goat weed can minimize fatigue and increase athletic performance

ix.   It helps to enrich skin health and also treat skin disease

x.   It aids to enrich hair growth

Some of the side effect you might experience when consume overdose of Horny goat weed are:

i.   It might cause nose bleeding

ii.   Excess sweating

iii.   It might lower your blood pressure

iv.   It might cause dry mouth.

v.   Dry mouth

What is Tribulus Terrestris?

Tribulus Terrestris which is also known as puncture vine is a flowering plant that belong to the family of

Zygophyllaceae. It is usually planted in a dry climate situated area in which a lot of plants can't survive and commonly found in Africa, Asia, Europe and Australia. Tribulus Terrestris is said to contribute to entire physical as such as sexual energy, cure bladder disorder, uro-genital and unitary tract conditions, used for treatment of all types of fever, increase testosterone level, libido, vitality, fertility and sperm motility in male. Tribulus Terrestris has been one of the vital constituent used in the making of supplement because of its potency to boost entire sexual performance in male and this actually the main reason why it was also added as one of the significant ingredient for the making of MEN'S SEXUAL ENRICHMENT FORMULA.

Some of its benefit of includes:

i.   It helps to reduce blood pressure by enriching the

heart

ii.   It helps to protect the blood vessel from damages cause as a result of high cholesterol diet

iii.   It can be used to treat erectile dysfunction to achieve enhanced sexual performance

iv.   It aids to increase your muscle frame and endurance level which on the other hand helps to improve athletic performance

v.   It aids to enrich mood

vi.   It aids the reduction of some type of cancer

vii.   It helps you to sustain and retain a tougher and long lasting erection

viii.   It increase your sexual self-confidence

ix.   Tribulus has an inflammatory properties

x.   Tribulus extract also helps to prevent calcium oxalate from producing and building up crystals in the kidney cell.

What is Pomegranate?

Pomegranate which is also known as anaar in hindi is a very sweet fruit with hard leathery skin on the outer layer and bunches of small edible red colored seed inside referred to as Arils. Scientifically it belong to the family of Lythraceae and it is usually used by the natives people of Persia, India, Asia and the Mediterranean region for wine making, juice blend, baking food species, and smoothies. It is generally used in Ayurveda to produce care for many disease because of the medical health potency contain in the arils. The arils are known to be a very good source of mineral, folic acid, vitamin A, C and E and also fiber.a research study also prove that the Pomegranate contain anti-oxidant action triple times higher than that of green tea or red wine.

Pomegranate is consider to have an advantageous effect on erectile dysfunction because it improve the Nitric oxide form in the body, this can actually aid the flow of blood to the penis for good erection and also assist the body to deliver additional oxygen to your body muscle tissue however increasing your energy and entire ability to function better with getting exulted.

Some of the benefit of Pomegranate includes:

i. When used it helps you to increase aerobic performance and also athletes endurance level

ii. It covert excess fat form in the body into muscle

iii. It enhances your level of energy to enable you carry out your regular activities, exercise and also help you with ability to recover loss energy on time

iv. It helps you to burn out to much weight gain

v. Pomegranate help to boost memory in adults

vi. It also help to minimize the risk of type two diabetes

vii. Pomegranate aid the support of anti-microbial abilities and your immune system

viii. Pomegranate helps to minimize the chances of cardiovascular disease

ix. Pomegranate carries an antioxidant properties that aid the blockage of the production of cartilage destroying enzyme

x. The superb fruit aid to lower high blood pressure

What is Ginkgo Biloba?

Ginkgo Biloba which is also referred to as Ginkgo which scientifically belong to the Ginkgoaceae family and only the surviving spices in the division of Ginkgophyta. It was first discover in the fossils two hundred and sixty years ago and it was cultivated initially in human history. This herbs is originally native to china and also has a history of been in use for decades currently now as traditional medicine to enhance health, sexual performance and brain in male and also use in the making of meal. Gingko functions as to enhance the release of oxygen in the human body; this takes place by breaching the platelets that help the flow of blood all over the body easily broadering the blood vessels that transport blood into the brain

Research Studies that is carried out on Ginkgo proves that it is qualify of relaxing blood pressure and improve vasodilatation, this can also aid to increase the flow of blood into the penile chamber for a longer period of time and better erection. All this can help to improve and boost your sexual functionalities in male with erectile dysfunction.

The benefit of Ginkgo Biloba are:

i.   It can be used for the treatment of erectile dysfunction

ii.   When taken it helps to enrich human memory & thinking

iii.   When taken it helps to ease the symptoms of anxiety, depression and stress

iv.   It can be used to boost human cognitive function

v.   Ginkgo Biloba can be used to enhance human sexual energy

vi.   Ginkgo Biloba can increase the vision of individual suffering from glaucoma

vii.   Ginkgo Biloba when taken it helps to boost your

sperm quality, libido and potency in male

viii. It energize you to be ever ready to perform excellently at any given task

ix. When taken it helps to increase the production of testosterone level in men body

x. When taken it helps to safeguard the nerves, your heart muscle and retina from damaging and also keep you safe from high blood pressure.

The expected side effect you might experience when using overdose Ginkogo bilola includes:

i. Having the symptoms of restlessness

ii. Having diarrhea

iii. Vomiting

iv. Experiencing dizziness

What is Panex Ginseng Root?

Panex Ginseng Root is the root of a plant also referred to as Panex Ginseng or Korean ginseng that usually grow in the Eastern Asia Mountain. This special of all plant belong to a scientific family called Araliaceae and it root is the actual source of ginseng which have many vitamins, mineral and nutrient. It is most time generally used in the making of supplement because of its remarkable healing properties, people usually prefer only the complete grown product because it is highly rich with healthy element.

Panex Ginseng is largely accepted as one of the unique herbs use for the treatment of men sexual dysfunction, enhancing sex hormone, boosting stamina and endurance level.

The benefit of Panex Ginseng are:

i.   When taken is helps to enrich your sex desire and

general mood

ii. When consume it helps to enhance your lean muscle mass by improving the nitric acid in your blood

iii. It heighten your mood and increase cognition

iv. When consume it helps to burn body and belly fat, helping you to recover the body physique you have always dream of

v. When consume it helps to enrich you immune system

vi. It is very rich with anti-aging properties

vii. When taken it helps you to boost your energy level

viii. When consume you stand to achieve an enhanced physical and sexual performance

ix. When taken it helps to boost the production of testosterone by improving the release of luteinizing hormone

x.   It helps to minimize high cholesterol from your body.

The expected side effect you may experience when you consume excess of Panex Ginseng includes:

i.   You may experience insomnia when consume too much

ii.   Symptoms of headache

iii.   Nervousness

iv.   Excess of Panex Ginseng may causes low blood sugar

What Is Zinc?

Zinc is a very significant component that helps you to live a very healthy also control the immune system in the body. Hence this component can't be generated by the body, it is very essential you ingest plenty amount of zinc because inadequate of zinc in the body might lead to zinc insufficiency which can affect your health harmfully.

Research has proven that zinc plays lots of vital roles in the body like: increasing the production of testosterone, treating of ED, triggers the deed of over 100 different enzymes in the body, absorb nutrients, generate protein, DNA and immune functions.

What are the symptoms Of Zinc deficiency?

Zinc deficiency actually means when the body lack the suppose amount of Zinc expected or required in a human body and this symptoms are:

i. Lack of adequate Zinc may lead to skin rash or disease

ii. Loss of appetite

iii.   Wound may take longer time to heal

iv.   Lack of adequate Zink in human body may causes loss of hair

v.   Lack of sufficient zinc in your body you may be experiencing blur vision

vi.   Inadequate Zinc in human body reproductive organs might get damage

vii.   Your sense of smell may fail

viii.   Lack of adequate Zinc may prompt to weaken immune system

ix.   Depression

x.   Digestion difficulty which can lead to constipation

The benefit of Zinc are:

i.   Sufficient zinc in your body helps you to increase

the level of testosterone production in your body

ii. Adequate zinc in human body helps to stabilize blood pressure

iii. Zinc ion the body helps to balance the hormonal system

iv. The body needs zinc to protect the skin from infection

v. Zinc help the body to be energetic as it boost your energy level

vi. Adequate Zinc in the body help to boost male potency and fertility

vii. Zinc in the body helps to minimize severe cold hay fever

viii. Adequate Zinc in your body help your wound to recover fast

ix.   It helps you to prevent any chances of memory loss

But then, high level of Zinc in the body can prompt to the following side effects:

i.   Vomiting

ii.   Allergies

iii.   Stomach disorder

iv.   headache

What types of food contain Zinc?

Food that are very rich in Zinc include:

i.   Pork lion

ii.   Yoghurt

iii.   Beefs

iv.   Pumpkin seeds

v.   Crabs and Lobster

vi.   Peanut

vii.   Beans

viii.   Baked beans

ix.   Oyster

x.   Peas

About The Book

MEN'S SEXUAL ENRICHMENT FORMULA" is a book written by Dr. Inks Swiss to guide you through why you really need this 100% natural male sex enrichment formula that is very helpful and effective in the prevention and treatment of different kind of erectile dysfunctions (ED) such as; premature ejaculation, low or poor libido, swing mood or sex urge, low stamina or poor endurance level etc. not just that but also help you to enlarge your penis to become bigger, thicker and harder to enjoy a long lasting erection.

Grab your copy and enjoy the best of your sexual lifestyle!

www.ingramcontent.com/pod-product-compliance
Lightning Source LLC
Chambersburg PA
CBHW051406150726
48000CB00003B/1350